SCOLIOSIS SURGERY RECOVERY DIET

Proven Surgical Techniques And Navigating Your Path To Healing For Reclaiming Strength And Healthy Lifestyle

DR LUCAS KAYCE

DISCLAIMER

This book about illness and nutrition is not meant to replace expert medical advice, diagnosis, or treatment; rather, it is meant purely for informational reasons. This book's content is founded on broad concepts and recommendations for managing diseases and nutrition.

Before adopting any major dietary or lifestyle changes, readers are recommended to speak with a qualified healthcare provider, such as a licensed physician or registered dietitian, especially if they have pre-existing medical concerns. Everybody has different health demands, so what works for one person might not work for another.

The use of the information provided in this book may have unfavorable repercussions or consequences, for which the author and publisher disclaim all liability. No disease is meant to be identified, treated, cured, or prevented by the information provided.

The book may include contain references to medical literature or research findings; however readers are urged to independently confirm this material and contact reliable sources.

It is important to remember that the fields of nutrition and medicine are always changing, and that new findings could have an impact on the advice offered in this book. As a result, readers are urged to keep up with the most recent advancements in healthcare and, when in doubt, seek professional counsel.

By reading this book, readers agree that they are in charge of their own health decisions and release the author and publisher from any liability arising from the use of the material in the book, whether direct or indirect.

TABLE OF CONTENTS

ABOUT THE BOOK

For those having scoliosis surgery, the book "Scoliosis Surgery Recovery Diet" is a vital resource that highlights the critical part that nutrition plays in the healing process. The first few chapters give a thorough overview of scoliosis, the surgical procedures associated with it, and the signs that call for surgery.

The importance of nutrition during the healing process is discussed, with a focus on the particular dietary requirements following surgery. This section explains how eating a balanced diet aids in the healing process, emphasizing the significance of dietary decisions made throughout the convalescence phase.

"Building a Foundation: Preparing for Surgery" provides helpful information on preoperative nutrition guidelines, suggested foods, and hydration techniques. This chapter focuses on creating the best possible environment for a successful recovery by addressing body preparation before surgery.

The ensuing chapters discuss various stages of the healing process. The early stages of recovery are discussed. Postoperative dietary guidelines, methods for controlling pain and inflammation with meals, and ideas for readily absorbed foods are all covered.

The importance of nutrient-rich foods is covered in detail, along with the vitamins, minerals, protein, and omega-3 fatty acids that are critical for the healing process. It also offers advice on how to include these nutrients in the meals that readers eat every day.

"Special Considerations for Dietary Restrictions", possible problems arising from dietary limits are discussed, along with recommendations for people with allergies or special dietary needs, such as veganism, vegetarianism, gluten-free, or dairy-free diets.

The book offers helpful advice on meal planning and recipe development, highlighting the significance of careful meal preparation during the healing process.

This contains nutrient-dense, simple-to-prepare recipes and sample meal plans for different stages of rehabilitation.

The significance of staying hydrated and the function of supplements are discussed. It discusses the importance of maintaining hydration while recovering and offers suggestions for supplements, taking into account any possible drug interactions.

The "Long-Term Dietary Guidelines" recommend introducing exercise into the healing process, keeping a healthy and balanced eating pattern, and making a gradual transition to a regular diet.

The book explores the psychological and emotional facets of recovery, including topics such as emotional eating, the significance of getting help and therapy, and developing mindful eating practices. This thorough handbook guarantees that readers are prepared to handle any emotional or psychological obstacles that may surface during this time, in addition to being knowledgeable on the medical aspects of healing.

COMPREHENDING SURGERY FOR SCOLIOSIS

In the realm of orthopedics, scoliosis—a medical disorder marked by an abnormal curvature of the spine—has raised a lot of concerns. This curvature frequently appears sideways, resulting in a three-dimensional malformation that can affect a person's movement, posture, and general quality of life. Surgery for scoliosis becomes necessary to stabilize and straighten the spine when the curvature gets severe and progressive. This introduction explores the definition, kinds of scoliosis, indications for surgical intervention, and an outline of the surgical methods involved in scoliosis surgery. It also digs into a thorough understanding of the field.

SCOLIOSIS DEFINITION AND TYPES

According to definitions, scoliosis is a medical disorder marked by an abnormal lateral curvature of the spine, frequently with associated rotation. Although it can happen at any age, the most typical time to diagnose this deviation from the spine's natural alignment is during adolescence. Even though the precise etiology of scoliosis is frequently still unknown, there are several possible explanations for it, including congenital anomalies, neuromuscular disorders, and idiopathic causes. For example, the most common type of scoliosis is idiopathic, which has no known cause. The age of onset, the underlying etiology, and the curvature patterns—both structural and non-structural—that affect treatment choices are used to categorize the various forms of scoliosis.

SURGERY FOR SCOLIOSIS INDICATIONS

The severity and progression of the spinal curvature determine whether or not scoliosis surgery is necessary. This is not a decision that is made lightly. A patient's age, skeletal maturity, degree of curvature, and the existence of concomitant symptoms like pain or respiratory impairment are the main determinants of the indications for scoliosis surgery. Generally, surgery is contemplated when the curvature exceeds a threshold, usually between 40 and 50 degrees, and when conservative measures such as bracing are unable to arrest the advancement. The surgeon also assesses the patient's general health to make sure they are a good candidate for the surgery.

SYNOPSIS OF PROCEDURES FOR SCOLIOSIS SURGERY

Scoliosis surgery includes a variety of operations intended to stabilize the deformity and fix the spine's aberrant curvature, halting additional deformity. The specifics of the scoliosis, such as the location and degree of curvature, along with the patient's age and general health, determine the surgical procedure to be used. Spinal fusion is a common surgical operation in which two or more vertebrae are fused to form a solid bone structure utilizing instrumentation and bone transplants. An alternative method is to stabilize and straighten the spine by inserting rods, screws, or other devices.

Additionally, less invasive methods have surfaced that provide shorter recovery times and smaller incisions.

Comprehending scoliosis surgery necessitates a thorough investigation of its description, the many kinds of scoliosis, the justifications for surgical intervention, and a synopsis of the numerous surgical techniques utilized. This multimodal approach emphasizes how difficult it is to treat scoliosis and how crucial it is to customize interventions to the particulars of each patient's situation.

CHAPTER ONE

THE SIGNIFICANCE OF DIET IN THE HEALING PROCESS AFTER SCOLIOSIS SURGERY

NEEDS FOR NUTRITION FOLLOWING SURGERY

Scoliosis surgery is a major medical procedure that needs to be carefully planned to guarantee a full recovery. Among these, diet is essential for promoting the body's recuperation after surgery. Following scoliosis surgery, there is an increase in tissue healing, immunological reaction, and metabolic activity in the body. Sufficient nutritional assistance becomes crucial for fulfilling the increased energy and nutrient requirements necessary for the best possible recovery.

The patient's capacity to follow a regular diet may be impacted by the particular difficulties that the post-surgery phase brings. If not treated early on, conditions including pain, decreased appetite, and altered digestive function can lead to nutritional deficiencies. Thus, an extensive post-operative care plan must recognize and cater to the unique nutritional requirements of patients recovering from scoliosis surgery.

DIET'S FUNCTION IN HEALING

An effective nutrition plan is essential for speeding up the healing process following scoliosis surgery. For example, muscle regeneration and tissue repair depend on proteins. Consuming enough high-quality protein sources, such as fish, eggs, lean meats, and legumes, can aid in the reconstruction of tissues that have been injured during surgery.

Consuming protein also helps prevent muscular atrophy and increase general strength, both of which are critical for recovery.

Adequate consumption of vitamins and minerals is essential for the immune system and bone health in addition to proteins. For example, bone mineralization—which is especially important in the setting of scoliosis surgery, where spinal structures may be affected—requires calcium and vitamin D.

To assist achieve these basic nutrient requirements, a diet high in fruits, vegetables, dairy products, and fortified plant-based alternatives can be consumed.

Additionally, although it's sometimes forgotten, staying hydrated is just as important to the healing process. Transport of nutrients, blood circulation, and general cellular activity are all supported by a well-hydrated body. Patients are recommended to continue drinking enough fluids because dehydration can make problems worse and impede healing.

ADVANTAGES OF A BALANCED DIET

After scoliosis surgery, there are several advantages to following a well-balanced diet that go beyond simple nutritional assistance. A nutrient-dense diet not only helps tissues heal physically but also enhances general health. In addition to helping patients restore strength and endurance—both essential for the rehabilitation process—good nutrition also plays a role in the restoration of energy levels.

Additionally, a balanced diet helps to lessen inflammation, which is a major issue after surgery. Anti-inflammatory foods, including the omega-3 fatty acids in walnuts, flaxseeds, and fish, can be included to help control inflammation and facilitate a quicker healing process.

Beyond the physical, diet has an impact on mental health as well. Following surgery, patients who are in pain, stressed, or anxious may discover that some nutrients—like those in whole grains and fruits—have a good effect on their mood and cognitive abilities. Thus, keeping a balanced diet addresses both the physical and psychological components of healing, providing a comprehensive approach to post-surgery rehabilitation.

A successful and thorough recovery process for patients undergoing scoliosis surgery depends on identifying and meeting their dietary needs.

CHAPTER TWO

LAYING THE GROUNDWORK AND GETTING READY FOR SURGERY

GUIDELINES FOR PREOPERATIVE NUTRITION

Preoperative dietary guidelines are essential for optimizing a patient's general health and supporting their body's ability to undergo the upcoming surgical treatment in the preoperative phase leading up to surgery. These suggestions include nutritional advice as well as measures for staying hydrated, all designed to put the patient in the best possible condition for a successful surgery and a speedy recovery.

ITEMS TO ADD TO YOUR PREOPERATIVE DIET

With an emphasis on preoperative nutrition, patients must follow certain recommendations to improve their nutritional state. In the weeks preceding surgery, a well-proportioned and nutrient-dense diet can help promote better wound healing, lower the risk of infection, and enhance overall recovery results.

The focus is often on limiting processed and sugary meals that may impair the body's capacity to recover and increasing the consumption of a range of healthy foods, such as fruits, vegetables, lean meats, and whole grains.

One of the most important parts of preparation is choosing what foods to include in the preoperative diet. Lean meats, fish, eggs, and dairy products are examples of high-protein diets that should be prioritized because proteins are essential for the immune system and tissue repair.

Incorporating complex carbs from whole grains also contributes to a longer-lasting energy source, and fruits and vegetables offer vital antioxidants, vitamins, and minerals that promote general health.

HYDRATION TECHNIQUES

Preoperative planning includes hydration methods as well because maintaining the right fluid balance is essential for good body function.

Improved tissue perfusion, organ function, and blood circulation are all dependent on adequate hydration and are crucial both during and after surgery. In the days preceding the surgery, patients are frequently encouraged to drink plenty of water and abstain from excessive coffee and alcohol consumption, as these can exacerbate dehydration.

Individual demands and medical conditions must be taken into account when discussing preoperative hydration. To reduce the possibility of difficulties during surgery, some patients can be given special instructions on fasting before the procedure. But it's important to stay hydrated during the allotted period. In certain situations, especially if the patient is fasting for an extended period, intravenous fluids may be given to make sure they are well hydrated.

Laying the groundwork for surgery requires a thorough approach to preoperative hydration and nutrition. Following certain instructions and including a diet that is well-balanced and full of vital nutrients can help people feel better overall and be more prepared for the upcoming surgery. Hydration techniques that are customized for each patient and take medical concerns into account help to ensure that the body is in the best possible condition for surgery and speed up the healing process.

CHAPTER THREE

DIETARY GUIDELINES FOR POSTOPERATIVE PATIENTS

The first recovery phase following surgery is a crucial time when the body starts to repair and rebuild strength. Dietary guidelines following surgery are essential for promoting this healing process. These suggestions frequently center on giving the body the nourishment it needs without placing an undue strain on the digestive system. To facilitate healing and avoid difficulties, you must adhere to the advice given by healthcare specialists.

Postoperative dietary guidelines usually recommend a diet high in nutrients and balanced. Since proteins are the building blocks of cells and are critical to the healing process, consuming an adequate amount of protein is necessary for tissue repair and recovery. In addition, consuming enough calories is necessary to fulfill the higher energy requirements linked to the healing process. Certain dietary adjustments, including avoiding particular foods or increasing fluid intake, may be advised depending on the type of operation and the patient's medical history.

USING DIET TO CONTROL PAIN AND INFLAMMATION

Another area that is frequently addressed during the initial phase of recovery is the management of pain and inflammation through food. Some foods have anti-inflammatory qualities that can help reduce pain and promote the body's natural healing processes. It has been demonstrated that foods high in omega-3 fatty acids, like walnuts, flaxseeds, and fatty fish, have anti-inflammatory properties. Consuming a diet rich in antioxidant-rich fruits and vegetables can also help to lower inflammation.

SOFT AND SIMPLE FOODS TO DIGEST

To reduce strain on the digestive system during the early stages of recuperation, soft, easily digested foods are typically advised. These foods are better for people who might have digestive discomfort after surgery since they are easier for the body to digest and softer on the stomach. Cooked grains, mashed potatoes, pureed soups, and thoroughly cooked veggies are a few examples of soft and easily digested foods. During this phase, meals that are spicy, greasy, or too fibrous should be avoided since they may be more difficult to digest and may cause irritation to the digestive tract.

Postoperative food guidelines are essential for promoting the first healing phase following surgery. A nutritious, well-balanced diet combined with mindful eating choices to reduce pain and inflammation can make a big difference in the healing process. Additionally, choosing foods that are soft and simple to digest reduces stress on the digestive system and frees up energy for the body to heal itself. Following these dietary recommendations in cooperation with medical professionals facilitates a quicker and more successful recovery process.

CHAPTER FOUR

RICH IN NUTRIENTS FOODS FOR HEALING

VITAL ELEMENTS FOR HEALING

The body's repair mechanisms are largely dependent on the critical nutrients that are consumed during the healing and recovery process. These nutrients are essential for boosting immune system function, encouraging tissue regeneration, and generally accelerating healing. Protein is one of the most important nutrients for healing and is considered the building block of nutrition.

PROTEIN

Because protein helps to rebuild and repair tissues, it is necessary for healing and recuperation. It is made up of amino acids, which are the building blocks of the body's muscles, organs, and other tissues. It's critical for those healing from illnesses, surgeries, or injuries to get enough protein.

Lean meats, chicken, fish, eggs, dairy products, legumes, and plant-based foods like tempeh and tofu are good sources of high-quality protein.

MINERALS AND VITAMINS

Micronutrients including vitamins and minerals have a variety of functions during the healing process. For example, the creation of collagen, a protein that serves as the structural basis for skin, bones, and connective tissues, depends on vitamin C. In the meantime, the immune system and wound healing are supported by minerals like copper and zinc. An ample supply of essential micronutrients is ensured by a balanced diet rich in fruits, vegetables, whole grains, and nuts, which supports a holistic approach to healing.

THE FATTY ACIDS OMEGA-3

Essential fats known as omega-3 fatty acids play a major role in the body's anti-inflammatory functions. While inflammation is a normal reaction to trauma, persistent inflammation can slow down the healing process. Walnuts, chia seeds, flaxseeds, and fatty fish like salmon and mackerel are good sources of omega-3 fatty acids. By incorporating these foods into their diet, people can reduce inflammation and create an environment that is more healing-friendly.

INCLUDING FOODS HIGH IN NUTRIENTS IN EVERYDAY MEALS

Developing a nutrient-rich diet that promotes healing requires planning each day's meals carefully. Making a variety of whole foods a priority guarantees a wide range of vital nutrients. An assortment of fruits and vegetables on a colorful platter offers a range of vitamins and minerals. Whole grains add extra vitamins and fiber, such as brown rice and quinoa. The body needs more protein during recuperation, so it's helpful to have lean proteins from both plant and animal sources.

Furthermore, as water is vital for many physiological functions, such as waste removal and nutrition delivery, it is imperative to pay attention to hydration.

Herbal broths and teas offer extra health advantages like antioxidants and can help increase fluid intake as well.

A comprehensive approach to nutrition is necessary on the path to healing and recovery. Important nutrients that promote the body's natural healing processes include protein, vitamins, minerals, and omega-3 fatty acids. Through the inclusion of diverse nutrient-dense foods in regular meals, people can enhance their dietary intake and provide a setting that supports prompt and efficient recuperation.

CHAPTER FIVE

PARTICULAR TAKEAWAYS FOR DIETARY LIMITATIONS

HANDLING ALLERGIES AND DIETARY RESTRICTIONS

In the hotel and food service industries, making accommodations for dietary needs and allergies is crucial to guarantee that every customer has a great and inclusive experience. Comprehending and executing specific dietary requirements not only signifies a dedication to meeting the needs of patrons but also enhances an establishment's overall standing. Recognizing and taking appropriate action in response to different dietary restrictions and allergies is one of the most important factors in this regard.

OPTIONS FOR VEGETARIANS OR VEGANS

As vegetarianism and veganism gain popularity, it is becoming more and more vital to cater to those who lead these lifestyles. While vegetarians refrain from eating any meat, poultry, or fish, vegans even go so far as to abstain from all animal products, such as dairy and eggs. Acknowledging the importance of these dietary choices, restaurants are expanding the range of plant-based options on their menus.

Offering vegetarian and vegan foods guarantees that a wider range of patrons can enjoy a fulfilling and inclusive eating experience. These recipes range from hearty vegetable-based dinners to inventive plant-powered alternatives.

This not only meets the increasing need for plant-based options but also demonstrates a dedication to inclusivity and diversity in the food industry.

DAIRY-FREE AND GLUTEN-FREE SUBSTITUTES

Common dietary issues like lactose intolerance and gluten intolerance necessitate careful consideration when choosing ingredients and preparing meals. Dairy-free diets exclude all dairy products, whereas gluten-free diets call for avoiding wheat, barley, and rye.

For example, people with gluten sensitivity or celiac disease, or those who are lactose intolerant or live a dairy-free lifestyle, require customized alternatives.

It is necessary to have a deep grasp of component composition and cross-contamination hazards to provide dairy-free and gluten-free alternatives.

To maintain the integrity of their gluten-free goods, establishments must source certified gluten-free grains, flour, and other ingredients. A more inclusive dining experience can also be achieved by developing dairy-free versions of well-known meals and providing dairy-free milk substitutes.

Managing dietary constraints and allergies in the kitchen is a dynamic process that involves ongoing awareness and adjustment. In addition to satisfying the dietary requirements of their diverse audience, food service enterprises show their dedication to culinary innovation and customer pleasure by offering vegetarian or vegan options, as well as gluten-free and dairy-free alternatives.

CHAPTER SIX

RECIPES AND MEAL PLANNING FOR THE RECOVERY AFTER SCOLIOSIS SURGERY

THE VALUE OF MEAL PREPARATION

Organizing meals is essential to promoting the healing process following scoliosis surgery. Gaining strength, controlling discomfort, and healing all depend on eating a healthy diet. A carefully planned diet makes sure that patients recovering from scoliosis surgery get the nutrients they need to speed up healing, lessen inflammation, and stay healthy overall.

Meal planning is crucial since it allows you to customize your diet to a patient's unique requirements while they heal from scoliosis surgery.

A balanced combination of vitamins and minerals helps strengthen the immune system and speeds up the healing process, while an adequate protein intake is essential for muscle repair and rebuilding. Given the effects of scoliosis surgery on the spine, it is especially crucial for bone health to include foods high in calcium and vitamin D.

EXAMPLE MEAL SCHEDULES FOR VARIOUS REHAB STAGES

It is vital to develop prototype meal plans for distinct stages of recuperation to cater to the changing nutritional needs during the therapeutic process. Soft, easily digested foods are advised during the first stages, while the body is still getting used to the surgical intervention. Soups, pureed veggies, and protein-packed smoothies may fall under this category. A progressive switch to more solid and varied foods can be made as the healing process advances, offering a greater variety of nutrients to aid in the healing process as a whole.

Meal planning for individuals should take into account their dietary choices, limitations, and any advice from medical professionals. A day in the early stages of recuperation, for instance, could consist of baked salmon with steamed vegetables for dinner, vegetable soup for lunch, and oatmeal for breakfast. Yogurt or fruit smoothies can be eaten as snacks in between meals.

SIMPLE TO MAKE AND PACKED WITH NUTRIENT RECIPES

Meal preparation following recovery from scoliosis surgery can be made easier with the help of nutrient-dense, easy-to-prepare meals. Quick and easy recipes ensure that patients' nutritional needs are satisfied without adding undue stress to them or their carers. Simple dishes like quinoa salad with veggies or roasted chicken with sweet potatoes may be both nutrient-dense and simple to prepare.

Pay special attention to adding foods high in anti-inflammatory components, like omega-3 fatty acids, which are present in nuts, seeds, and seafood. Furthermore, a range of vitamins and antioxidants may be found in colored fruits and vegetables, which can improve general health. Playing around with herbs and spices can add flavor to food without sacrificing nutritional value, especially when taking into account any changes in appetite or taste preferences during the healing process.

Food planning is essential to the healing process following scoliosis surgery. It guarantees that people get the proper nutrients at every turn during their recuperation, promoting bone health, muscle growth, and general well-being. Customized sample meal plans and simple, nutrient-dense meals are crucial components that make the healing process go more smoothly and successfully.

CHAPTER SEVEN

DRINKING WATER AND TAKING SUPPLEMENTS

HYDRATION IS ESSENTIAL FOR RECOVERY

When it comes to recuperation, especially after physical activity and exercise, hydration is essential. Sustaining the body's general health and functionality requires proper hydration. Sweating causes the body to lose fluids during exercise, thus it's important to replace these lost fluids to avoid dehydration.

Numerous negative outcomes, such as diminished performance, cramping in the muscles, and an elevated risk of heat-related disorders, can result from dehydration.

Adequate hydration facilitates the effective delivery of nutrients to cells throughout the healing process, supporting the reconstruction and restoration of tissues that may have been strained or damaged during physical exertion.

Moreover, enough hydration promotes body temperature regulation and joint lubrication, all of which aid in a quicker and more efficient healing process.

SUGGESTED ADD-ONS

Supplementation, when combined with adequate hydration, can be an important part of an all-encompassing recovery plan. Athletes and people who exercise vigorously should think about taking specific supplements to help with their general health and performance.

The majority of nutrients must come from a balanced diet, however, supplements can help close any nutritional gaps and speed up healing. Supplements that are frequently advised include protein, which promotes muscle growth and repair; branched-chain amino acids (BCAAs), which are well-known for their ability to lessen muscle soreness; and electrolytes, which are essential for preserving appropriate fluid balance and avoiding dehydration.

When used as directed, these supplements can aid in a quicker recovery and better physical health in general.

MEDICATIONS AND POSSIBLE INTERACTIONS

It is imperative to acknowledge the possibility of supplement and medicine interactions. Some supplements have the potential to have unexpected results by interfering with the medication's effectiveness or absorption. For example, vitamin K may interact with blood-thinning drugs, and calcium supplements may prevent some antibiotics from being absorbed. Before adding supplements to their regimen, people should always speak with healthcare providers, especially if they are on prescription drugs.

By doing this, possible interactions are recognized and handled properly, avoiding any negative health impacts. Establishing a safe and efficient supplementing plan that supports overall healing efforts requires open communication between patients and healthcare providers.

Staying hydrated is essential to the healing process since it helps to sustain biological processes, facilitates the transfer of nutrients, and guards against problems brought on by dehydration. As you're thinking about supplements for your recovery plan, pay special attention to well-studied choices like protein, BCAAs, and electrolytes.

CHAPTER EIGHT

LONG-TERM DIETARY
RECOMMENDATIONS

PROGRESSIVE SWITCH TO A REGULAR DIET

One of the most important components of long-term dietary guidelines is the gradual shift to a regular diet, especially following a time of food restriction or therapeutic interventions. This method reduces the possibility of stomach discomfort or other negative reactions by acknowledging the significance of letting the body adjust to changes gradually. Whether regaining health after an illness, managing weight, or correcting dietary inadequacies, a gradual return to a variety of food categories can support long-term well-being.

This gradual shift takes into account each person's tolerances and preferences while acknowledging the importance of patience and awareness. It frequently entails a step-by-step process in which foods that may have been limited are progressively introduced while the body is constantly monitored for any reactions. This promotes psychological health in addition to helping with physical adjustment and cultivates a healthy relationship with food. The objective is to create a pleasurable and long-lasting eating routine that supports long-term health objectives.

KEEPING A BALANCED AND HEALTHFUL DIET

Eating a healthy, balanced diet is the cornerstone of long-term dietary advice. The significance of eating a range of nutrient-dense meals that supply important vitamins, minerals, and other key nutrients is emphasized by this principle. A variety of fruits, vegetables, nutritious grains, lean meats, and healthy fats are usually found in a balanced diet. Finding the ideal balance guarantees that the body gets the nutrients it needs to function at its best, enhancing general health and well-being.

Furthermore, moderation and conscious portion control are essential to maintaining a balanced diet.

This strategy permits infrequent indulgences while assisting in preventing overconsumption of particular food groups. A healthy diet must include adequate water as well because it supports several body processes and increases general vitality. Following these dietary guidelines for an extended period helps maintain energy levels, boost immune system performance, and lower the chance of developing chronic illnesses.

INCLUDING EXERCISE IN THE PROCESS OF RECOVERY

Long-term dietary advice must include frequent exercise as part of the rehabilitation process. Maintaining a healthy weight and improving general health are greatly aided by physical activity. Exercise supports a holistic approach to well-being by enhancing muscular strength, flexibility, and cardiovascular health. Exercise regimens specifically designed for specific goals such as weight loss, chronic condition management, or injury recovery increase the efficacy of dietary therapies.

Exercise improves mental and physical health in addition to physical health. Frequent exercise has been associated with lowered stress levels, happier moods, and better cognitive performance. Exercise regimens and intensities might differ depending on a person's ability and health, which highlights the value of individualized and long-term strategies. Combining exercise with a healthy diet works in concert to support a holistic approach to long-term health and energy during the recovery process.

CHAPTER NINE

ASPECTS OF RECOVERY THAT ARE PSYCHOLOGICAL AND EMOTIONAL

HANDLING EMOTIONAL EATING

Emotional eating is a complicated issue that is closely related to a person's psychological and emotional health. It frequently acts as a coping technique for handling stress, worry, or other difficult feelings. Understanding and treating emotional eating is a critical component of the healing process.

People can learn more effective coping strategies by comprehending the feelings and triggers that underlie the desire to eat. Developing self-awareness and mindfulness is necessary to differentiate between emotional desires and physical hunger.

Building a healthy connection with food and discovering healthy coping mechanisms for emotions is critical during the healing process.

SEEKING COUNSELING AND SUPPORT

When it comes to the emotional and psychological components of rehabilitation, it is not advisable to go it alone. Navigating the challenges of rehabilitation requires seeking out counseling and assistance. Making a connection with a mental health expert or participating in support groups gives people a secure forum to share their ideas and emotions. Through the exploration of the underlying reasons for emotional suffering, therapy sessions can assist individuals in developing efficient coping mechanisms. Talking openly and honestly with a therapist or in a community of support creates a sense of empowerment, understanding, and affirmation that aids in emotional healing and resilience.

PRACTICES OF MINDFUL EATING

Mindful eating is an all-encompassing strategy that promotes people to develop presence and awareness during meals. This technique entails being aware of one's hunger and fullness cues in addition to focusing on the sensory qualities of eating, such as flavor, texture, and aroma. Using mindful eating techniques can greatly improve people's emotional and psychological health when they are in recovery. People can improve their relationship with food and make dining a more purposeful and fulfilling experience by taking their time and enjoying every bite. By promoting a non-judgmental awareness of thoughts and feelings connected to food, mindful eating also helps people eat more healthily and have a better relationship with themselves.

Treating emotional eating, getting help and counseling, and implementing mindful eating techniques are essential elements of the psychological and emotional aspects of recovery.

www.ingramcontent.com/pod-product-compliance
Lightning Source LLC
Chambersburg PA
CBHW060815260726
48660CB00002B/953